SANKOFA HERBAL REMEDIES

RECIPE BOOK
FOR GENERAL HEALTH

Foreword

This book contains simple remedies to keep the body strong and ward off the onset of a whole host of serious diseases and health issues.

The herbs contained herein are those required for everyday ailments for cure or prevention for the body.

By following and taking a few of the remedies here once a week, your life will be healthy and happy. Extensive reading on the herbs is also recommended as they may offer remedies to more ailments than are not listed here.

Consult your doctor too if you do have any serious ailments that will interact adversely with the herbs or affect your health if you do. Pregnant or breastfeeding mothers should also consult their doctors before taking herbs.

Most of the herbs mentioned are for preventative purposes and to have general health and prevent **DIS~EASE**.

SOURSOP LEAVES

People in Africa and South America use the bark, leaves, root, and fruits of the graviola tree for general healthy remedies.

In laboratory studies, graviola extracts have been validated to kill some types of liver and breast cancer cells. These cells are resistant to some chemotherapy drugs.

Many sites on the internet advertise and promote graviola capsules as a cancer cure. It depletes and removes mucus from the body which is the most common causes of illness these days. Taking this leaf drink once a week will prevent a lot of diseases that is why it was stated here first.

Diseases it can fight against are:

- Kills a wide spectrum of viruses (including HIV)
- Kills parasites in the body
- Reduces rheumatism
- Cures arthritis
- Removes excess phlegm and mucus from the body
- Cleanses the blood
- Kills a wide spectrum of cancer cells
- Kills liver cancer cells and cleanses the liver
- Kills breast cancer cells
- Kills prostrate cancer cells

Direction

1. Dry the leaves indoors so they are dried but green
2. Boil 5 or 10 leaves in double the water amount until red and the water reduces to half the amount before boiling
3. Drink 1 cup morning and evening. Add lime, honey or turmeric if desired.
4. To be taken 1cup a day until feeling better. 1 cup every 2 weeks drank over 2 days is good for general health.

LEMON GRASS LEAVES

Lemongrass might help prevent the growth of some bacteria and yeast. It is also used to kill germs and as a mild astringent and it is good for cleansing the bloodstream.

Diseases it can fight against are:

- Pain in the nerves from swelling like GOUT
- Reduce Fever
- Improve levels of sugar and cholesterol in the blood
- Stimulate the uterus and menstrual flow
- Has antioxidant properties
- Treating digestive tract spasms
- Helps cure stomach ache and pains
- Reduces high blood pressure
- Treats convulsions, pain and vomiting
- Reduces coughs
- Drains achy joints (Rheumatism)
- Treat fever and common cold
- Exhaustion
- Cleanses the blood

Direction

1. Boil 1 teaspoon or more of the lemongrass tea for about 5 minutes. Sieve and drink. You can add honey
2. You can take the decoction once a week for general health

AGARICUS (Mushrooms)

This mushroom contains amylase, trypsin, maltase and protease. These enzymes assist the body to break down protein, carbohydrates and fats.

Diseases it can fight against are:

- Fights cancer tumour growth
- Type 2 diabetes
- Lowers high cholesterol
- Hardening of the arteries (arteriosclerosis)
- Ongoing Liver disease
- Bloodstream disorders
- Digestive problems
- Heart disease prevention
- Weakened bones (osteoporosis)
- Stomach and duodenal ulcers, chronic gastritis, constipation
- Viral enteritis, stomatitis
- Pyorrhea
- Strengthens immune system
- Works as an antioxidant
- Longevity of life when consumed on a regular basis

Direction

1. Powder, add a teaspoon to water or juice and drink every 3 days. It can also be added to food, sauces, soups to drink in moderation every couple of days.
2. Few drops(tincture) can be added to water and taken daily

Reishi (Mushrooms)

Mushroom containing active particles which boosts the brain, cardiovascular and immune system.

Contains polysaccharides and triterpenes which reduce inflammation in the body. The anti-inflammatory compounds in it inhibits histamine (the chemical responsible for allergic reactions) thereby decreasing the symptoms of allergies.

Diseases it can fight against are:
- Sleep disorders
- Anxiety attacks
- Depression
- Helps focus
- Weight loss
- Immune system booster
- Enhances liver health

Direction
1. Few drops(tincture) can be added to water and taken daily
2. Powder, add a teaspoon to water or juice and drink every 3 days. Can also be added to food, sauces, soups to drink in moderation every couple of days.

Chaga Mushroom

Diseases it can fight against are:
- Combats Aging (caused by oxidative stress)
- Inflammation
- Lowering LDL(low density lipoprotein aka bad cholesterol)
- Powerful antioxidant for fighting free radicals
- Bloodstream disorders
- Digestive problems

Direction
1. Powder, add a teaspoon to water or juice and drink every 3 days. It can also be added to food, sauces, soups to drink in moderation every couple of days.
2. Boil or prepare with soup to eat

Turkey Tail Mushroom

Diseases it can fight against are:

- Immune system booster
- Contains powerful antioxidants
- Helps fight certain cancers
- Improves Gut bacteria balance
- Brain booster
- Bloodstream disorders
- Digestive problems
- Powerful antioxidant for fighting free radicals

Direction

1. Powder, add a teaspoon to water or juice and drink every 3 days.
2. It can also be added to food, sauces, soups to drink.
3. Boil or prepare with soup to eat

Wormwood Plant (artemisinin)

Referred to as the "bitter plant", it has a long history of traditional use. Can be added to smoothies and drinks or if raw, boiled and drank as tea. Not to be consumed for 4-5 weeks straight.

Diseases it can fight against are:

- Loss of appetite
- Upset stomach
- Gall bladder disease
- Intestinal Spasms
- Treat fever
- Liver disease
- Depression
- Muscle pain
- Memory loss
- Worm infections
- Increase sexual desire
- Tonic
- To stimulate sweating

Direction

To be boiled and drank as tea when suffering from fever or other ailments listed. A teaspoon of it.

Can be drank a cup every 2 weeks for general health.

Holy Thorn Tea (Espintheira Santa or Chuchuhuasi)
Long history of use in South American herbalism. Regarded as a holy herb in indigenous folk healing practices.
Diseases it can fight against are:

- Decoction can decrease nervousness
- Supports digestive health
- Increase milk production
- Regulate high blood pressure
- Analgesic and anti-inflammatory
- Immune system booster
- Soothes gastrointestinal discomfort
- Decrease blood fats
- Used to treat heart failure
- Ease labour
- Promotes overall well-being

Direction
1. Soak the tea bag in hot water for a few minutes before drinking.
2. If chipped bark, boil 1-2 teaspoon of the bark, allow to steep for a few minutes and sieve to drink

Maca Powder

This herb is an ancient Peruvian superfood classed as an adaptogen.

It contains anthocyanins which enhances physical and mental performance.

Diseases it can fight against are:

- Increases libido
- Boosting energy and endurance
- Increase fertility and male reproductive health
- Improve mood
- Reduce blood pressure
- Reduce sun damage
- Fight free radicals

Direction

1. 1-3 teaspoons a day once per week
2. Powder can be sprinkled on porridge or added to tea, juice, warm or cold water. Milk and honey can be added to enhance flavour.

Muira Puama

Energy tonic in Brazilian and Latin American herbal folklore. Rich in EFA's (essential fatty acids), plant sterols and beta-sitosterol.

Diseases it can fight against are:

- Applied to cure alopecia
- Upset stomach
- Menstrual disorders
- Rheumatism
- Paralysis caused by Polio
- General tonic and appetite stimulant
- Helps with healthy ageing
- Aphrodisiac

Direction

1. When suffering from any of the ailments listed. Take 4 a day (2 in the morning and 2 at night) every 3 days.
2. Can be taken 2 every 2 weeks for general health

Hercampuri (for weight loss)

A wild plant that grows in the Andean mountainous regions. It's bitter leaves have been used for years to maintain stable cholesterol levels.

Diseases it can fight against are:

- Stomach pain
- Reduces and maintains cholesterol levels
- Combat malaria fever
- Restore hepatic functions
- Reduce obesity

Direction

1. Herbal tea to be put in boiled hot water, simmer for a few minutes and drink once or twice a week for general health.
2. When sick from any of the ailments above, drink a cup morning and evening till cured or symptoms subside

Carqueja Plant or Tea

A native plant found throughout South America. Research has shown the plant has antioxidant activity in vitro, as well as anti-inflammatory, antidiabetic, analgesic and antimutagenic properties.

Diseases it can fight against are:

- Treat pain and reduces fever
- Indigestion and constipation
- Swelling and water retention
- Constipation
- Protect the liver
- Prevent ulcers
- Purify the blood and poor circulation
- Regulates blood pressure and blood sugar
- Not for pregnant or lactating women

Direction

Tea to be taken when suffering from indigestion, constipation or after a heavy meal or few times a week.

Milk Thistle

A very important herb that has been curatively used for more than 2000 years. Has been used in ayurvedic medicine, in Latin America and in Europe for 1000 years to combat most of the ailments below.

Diseases it can fight against are:

- Kidney cleanse and repair
- Liver tonic. Restores liver from alcohol abuse, hepatitis, drug addiction
- A galactogogue: promotes lactation
- Cholagogue: stimulates flow of bile from the liver
- Anti fibrotic: prevents tissue scarring
- Prevents toxins getting into liver cells
- Counters nausea from alcohol and cirrhosis
- Contains antioxidants (glutathione and super oxide dismutase
- Glutathione protects intestines from inflammatory damage
- Silymarin improves blood and urine markers associated with diabetic kidney disease
- Helps enzyme formation, increases bile production from the liver
- Protects the mucus membranes

Direction

1. Take half teaspoon every once or twice a week and after drinking heavily or during hangover
2. Can be taken once every 2 weeks for general health for heavy drinkers to preserve liver health and chronic damage over time
3. Can be added to water or fruit juice. For tincture, 1-2ml at a time up to 3 times a day (not recommended in high doses as it has a laxative effect when consumed in high doses)

Artichoke

Artichoke is a part of the thistle biological family that are famous in use in detoxifying the body, especially the liver. It contains **Cynarin** which has many health benefits. Contains **Inulin** which can improve insulin resistance in people with type 2 diabetes.

Diseases it can fight against are:

- Detoxifying the body
- Improving and enhancing liver health and function
- Used to treat jaundice and hepatitis
- Used to stimulate flow of bile from liver and gall bladder to combat diabetes symptoms
- Used to treat heart conditions
- Helps accelerate liver regeneration and protect it from toxins
- Inulin helps balance microflora and good probiotic bacteria in the stomach
- Probiotics helps break down food in the stomach and eliminate toxins
- Helps relieve diarrhoea and constipation by normalising bowel movements
- Herb is rich in inulin (allows sugar to be released slowly into the body thereby promoting healthy blood sugar levels). A stool softener also.
- High in Vitamin B1 which help maintain healthy levels of hydrochloric acid in the stomach
- Rich in potassium to help normalise blood pressure by neutralising excess sodium in the body
- Cynarin also normalises cholesterol levels thereby lowering probability of stroke or heart attack

Direction

1. Can be drank as a tea which can be drank as often as possible.
2. For the leaves or powder, Infuse 1-2 teaspoons of Artichoke Leaf per cup of boiling hot water.
   Let the tea brew for 5 to 15 minutes. Strain and enjoy up to 3 times per day.

Burdock Root

This herb forms an important part in aiding the body's inner lymphatic drainage system rid the body of toxins. It is one of those herbs that can stimulate lymphatic drainage and detoxification. Also contains inulin to aid digestion.

Diseases it can fight against are:

- Soothing cleanse for kidneys, blood purifier. Stimulates bile production to help the liver flush away toxins.
- Relieving lymphatic system in body's inner drainage system
- Reduces rheumatic pains and aches
- Soothes gout pain
- Diuretic to stimulate kidneys to pass more urine
- Soothe stomach ailments
- Constipation and catarrh
- Alleviates fever and infection
- Fluid retention and skin problems
- Diaphoretic :promotes sweating
- Inulin helps improve digestion and remove toxins
- Contains mucilage to protect gastric mucosa(mucus membrane in the stomach)
- Contains antioxidants: quercetin, luteolin, phenolic acids
- Lowers inflammation and arthritis
- Helps fight acne and eczema in skin and promotes younger looking skin
- Beneficial for clearing and protecting the liver against poisonous substances.

Direction

1. A typical dosage of Burdock Root Powder is one to two grams of powdered dry root up to three times per day.
2. Burdock Root can be made into a herbal Tea. 1-2 teaspoons per cup of boiling water and steep for 3-10 minutes.
3. Tincture is traditionally taken 2-3ml, 2-3 times per day or as directed by a Herbal Practitioner.

Pau D'Arco

One of the most powerful herbs on the planet. Can be found mostly in Latin America.

Diseases it can fight against are:

- Cold, insect bites and fungal infections
- Skin infections, snake bites and impetigo
- Cures candida and thrush infections
- Loosen bowels and wash out old faecal matter
- Has anti- inflammatory properties
- Increases Nrf2 genes in intestines which protects against oxidative damage in the intestine
- Antioxidant/Antiviral: contains quercetin, flavonoids and carnosol
- Inhibits dangerous viruses like HIV from multiplying through beta-lapochone content which inhibits enzymes in virus cells
- Virus cannot take control of the reproductive process of the cell and can neither replicate or infect other cells

Direction

1. Tincture:
   For children up to 10 years- One and half of adult dose
   For children 14 years and up – Three quarters of adult dose
2. For Adults: 2-3ml; 2 - 3 times a day in water or juice.
3. Decoction: Boil 1 - 1½ tsp in 1 cup water for about 10 minutes. Drink 1 cup 2 - 3 times a day.
4. For general health, quarter teaspoon every 2 weeks.

Warning
(Very toxic when consumed in high doses and could lead have lethal consequences)

St Johns Wort

A remedy for mild to severe depression. Contains hypericin and hyperforin which are active ingredients for depression treatment medication. Lowers levels of stress and makes serotonin and dopamine to the brain.

Diseases it can fight against are:

- Mild to severe depression
- OCD (Obsessive Compulsive Disorder)
- PMS
- Nerve damage healing
- Damaged brain cell healing

Direction

1. Tincture: 2-4mls up to 3 times a day
2. Herbal Powder: 1-2 grams up to 3 times a day
3. Cut leaf (dried) or tea: 1-2 teaspoon per cup of boiling water. Simmer for 5 mins and drink up to 3 times a day

Hypoxis (African Potato)

Hypoxis hemerocallidea is a native plant that grows in the Southern African regions and is well known for its beneficial medicinal effects in the treatment of diabetes, cancer, and high blood pressure. Also contains sitosterol or phytosterol, an immune enhancer.

Diseases it can fight against are:

- Keep diabetes in check
- Prevents multiplication of cancer cells
- Used to build up the immune system of HIV sufferers
- Reduces high blood pressure
- Contains hypoxoside – a compound that is converted to rooperol which aids in fighting against inflammation, HIV and cancer cells in patients with these ailments
- Used to treat prostrate hypetrophy and urinary tract infections
- Used to shrink testicular tumours
- Laxative to expel intestinal worms
- Used to treat anxiety and heart palpitations
- Used to treat rheumatoid arthritis

Direction

1. Tincture : Add two or three drops to juice or water on an empty stomach and eat after 30 mins
2. Quarter tea spoon of powder or 2 to 3 drops of tincture added to drink once every week for general health.

Other varieties namely the H Colchicifolia and H Vilosa are toxic to humans and should not be consumed. Check the plant is H Hemerocallidea

Buchu Leaves

This is the best herb for treating urinary tract infections. Contains diosphenol a diuretic for urinary tract health. This flushes out harmful toxins from the body.

Diseases it can fight against are:

- Bladder health
- Increases fluid flow through kidneys
- Water retention, detoxifying agent
- Aids digestive Health
- Aids Blood Circulation
- Strengthen blood vessels (Rutin) in the heart muscles and arteries
- Soften and reduces varicose Veins
- Softens and reduces spider veins
- Cleanses digestive tract
- Anti spasmodic properties: helps relieve nausea, indigestion and flatulence
- Helps relieve and treats cystitis, urethritis and bladder irritation
- Dissolves and flushes out uric acid crystals from gout thereby making it potent to use during flares.

Direction

1. Tincture: 2-3ml taken 2-3 times per day,

2. Buchu Leaf Tincture can be added to water or fruit juice and taken when required.

Precautions

Buchu must not be consumed by pregnant women as it may stimulate the uterus. Not recommended for breastfeeding mothers.

Do not use Buchu 2 weeks before or after scheduled surgery. If you are suffering from acute kidney infection or liver disease, do not use this herb unless recommended by your healthcare practitioner.

Not recommended for pregnant or breastfeeding women.

Do not use Buchu 2 weeks before or after scheduled surgery. May cause stomach irritation. If you are suffering from acute kidney infection or liver disease, do not use this herb unless recommended by your healthcare practitioner.

Saw Palmetto

This is a plant found in North America and is renowned for its effective ability to protect against and treat the prostrate gland.

Diseases it can fight against are:

- Reduces or prevents prostrate from enlargement
- Alleviates urinary problems caused by an enlarged prostrate
- Reduces inflammation in the bladder of both men and women
- Amphoteric adaptogen- normalises reproductive functions in both men and women
- Improve sperm count in men
- Helps regularise hormonal imbalance in women
- As a result of improving urination, it empties the bladder thereby reducing kidney stones and kidney infections

Direction

1. **Tincture:** Take 1-2ml up three times a day
2. **Herbal Powder:** 1/3 - 2/3 grams
   up to 3 times a day or as directed by a herbalist

Do not combine with anti-androgenic medication.

Mutamba

Also known as West Indian Elm or Bay Cedar, this plant is good for stomach ailments, worms and mucus related maladies like HIV.

Diseases it can fight against are:

- Remedy for hair loss and baldness
- Reduces mucus in HIV sufferers and boosts immune system
- Digestive aid for stomach ache, diarrhoea, dysentery and stomach inflammation.
- Prevents ulcer
- Kills bacteria, fungal cells and cancer cells
- Cleanses blood, fights free radicals
- Stops bleeding, heals wounds
- Supports healthy heart functioning
- Suppresses coughs and relaxes muscles
- Protects and cleanses liver
- Reduces fever and inflammation
- Promotes perspiration

Direction

1. Bark Infusion – 1 cup, 1-3 times daily.
2. Capsules – 2 grams twice daily
3. Tincture – 2-3ml twice daily
4. For general health – Any of the above once a week

Epilogue

All people in our modern day and time do not take their general health seriously in what we eat, drink, do as well as exercise until we experience dis-ease. The herbs mentioned here taken in small and safe quantities can and will ensure that our bodies prevent the onset of diseases.

The simplicity of the publication is to get straight to the point of the anomalies the herbs treat instead of giving a thorough research on their history and origins. That can be investigated by the user when they are better and can understand the importance of simple herbal infusions weekly to help the body stay fit and healthy for years to come.

May the reader experience health and vitality and kindly send your views to **adofofelix@hotmail.com**. The author will appreciate your comments and hope this book will help keep you healthy till old age.

www.ingramcontent.com/pod-product-compliance
Lightning Source LLC
Chambersburg PA
CBHW081005290526
45795CB00009B/3083